NOURISHING HOPE

A Cancer-Fighting Diet Cookbook.

NITA P. AMOS

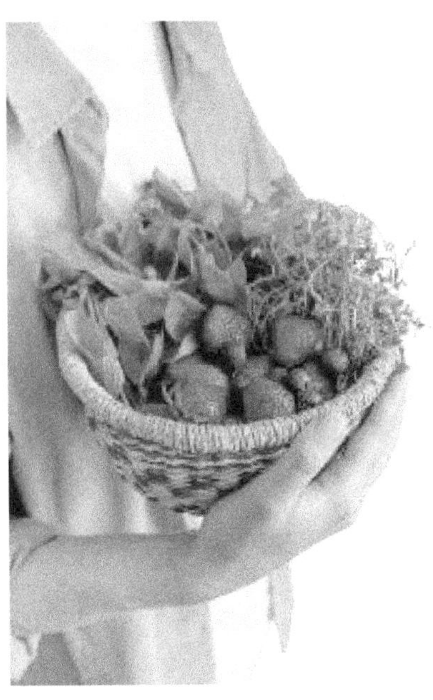

Copyright © 2024 by Nita P. Amos

All rights reserved.

Other books by Nita P. Amos

- <u>Savoring Life: A Journey through the Art of Eating</u>
- Nourishing Harmony: A Guide to Healing Foods for Optimal Health
- <u>20 Healthy Low Budget Recipes</u>

TABLE OF CONTENTS

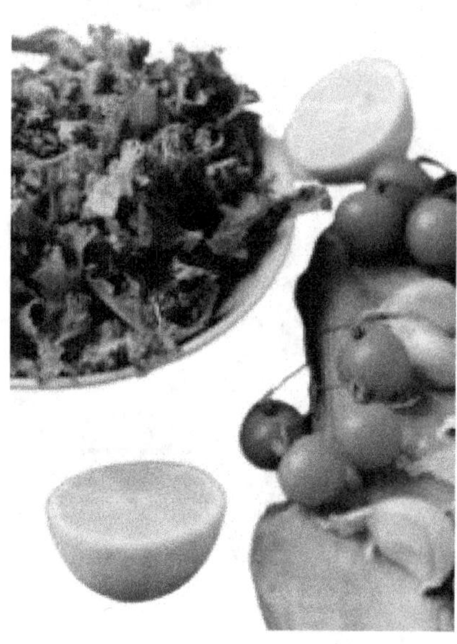

INTRODUCTION

In the delicate dance between life's fragility and the resilient human spirit, "Nourishing Hope: A Cancer-Fighting Diet Cookbook" emerges as a beacon of strength, sustenance, and the profound belief in the transformative power of nourishment. Within these pages, we embark on a journey that transcends the conventional boundaries of culinary exploration; it is a journey intertwined with the threads of courage, resilience, and the unwavering belief that every morsel can be a source of healing.

As we face the formidable adversary that is cancer, the kitchen becomes a sanctuary, a space where ingredients transform into allies, and each recipe is a testament to the human capacity to find hope amidst adversity. This cookbook is more than a collection of sumptuous dishes; it is a symphony of flavors harmonized with the gentle notes of compassion, science, and the unyielding belief that the right nourishment can be a formidable force in the face of the toughest battles.

"Nourishing Hope" is an ode to the indomitable spirit that refuses to succumb to despair, recognizing the profound impact a carefully curated diet can have on the intricate tapestry of wellness. It beckons us to embrace a cancer-fighting journey with joy, savoring the process of selecting, preparing, and relishing every bite as an act of self-love and resilience.

Here, each recipe is not merely a culinary creation; it is a gesture of love, a whisper of encouragement, and a beacon of light for those navigating the challenging path of cancer. From the vibrant hues of nutrient-dense salads to the comforting embrace of warm soups, each chapter encapsulates the promise of nourishment as a source of hope, vitality, and a tribute to the triumph of the human spirit.

Let "Nourishing Hope" be your companion, a guide infused with hope, wisdom, and the transformative power of a cancer-fighting diet. May this culinary journey illuminate your path, offering sustenance not only to the body but also to the soul, as we embrace the beauty and resilience inherent in every step towards healing.

CHAPTER 1

UNDERSTANDING NUTRITION AND CANCER.

Navigating a cancer diagnosis can be overwhelming, but understanding the crucial role that nutrition plays in supporting your body during this challenging time is a powerful step towards overall well-being.

Cancer and nutrition are intricately linked, with dietary choices playing a crucial role in both prevention and support during treatment.

Key principles to grasp include:

Balanced Diet:

- ❖ Prioritize a healthy diet rich in fruits, vegetables, whole grains, and lean meats.
- ❖ Ensure a variety of nutrients to support overall health.

Antioxidants and Phytochemicals:

- ❖ Include foods high in antioxidants (berries, leafy greens) and phytochemicals.

❖ These compounds combat oxidative stress and may help reduce cancer risk.

Healthy Fats:

❖ Choose sources of healthy fats including avocados, almonds, and olive oil.

❖ Omega-3 fatty acids, found in fish and flaxseeds, may have anti-inflammatory effects.

Limit Processed Foods:

❖ Minimize processed and red meat intake.

❖ Excessive consumption may contribute to cancer risk.

Hydration:

❖ Stay adequately hydrated to support bodily functions, especially during treatment.

❖ Water aids digestion and helps maintain energy levels.

Maintain a Healthy Weight:

❖ Achieving and maintaining a healthy weight is essential.

❖ Obesity is linked to an increased risk of certain cancers.

Individualized Approach:

❖ Recognize the uniqueness of each person's nutritional needs.
❖ Consult a healthcare expert or nutritionist for specific advice.

During Treatment:

❖ Cancer treatments may impact appetite and digestion.
❖ Focus on easily digestible, nutrient-dense foods.

Supplements:

❖ Consult healthcare professionals before taking supplements.
❖ Certain vitamins and minerals may require careful monitoring during cancer treatment.

Listen to Your Body:

❖ Pay attention to how certain meals make you feel.

❖ Adapt your diet based on individual tolerances and preferences.

Consult Healthcare Professionals:

❖ Collaborate with oncologists, dietitians, and nutritionists.

❖ They can provide tailored advice based on treatment plans and individual health status.

Community Support:

❖ Seek support from community groups or nutrition-focused programs.

❖ Sharing experiences and tips with others undergoing similar challenges can be valuable.

Understanding nutrition's role in cancer involves adopting a holistic approach, addressing both prevention and supportive care. By making informed dietary choices, individuals can positively impact their well-being and enhance their resilience during the cancer journey.

CHAPTER 2

BREAKFAST BOOSTERS

Breakfast is the cornerstone of your day, providing essential energy and nutrients to kickstart your morning. During your journey through cancer, a nourishing breakfast becomes even more critical. This chapter is dedicated to delicious and nutrient-dense breakfast options designed to fuel your body and set a positive tone for the day ahead.

SECTION 1: SMOOTHIE SENSATIONS:

1.1 Berry Blast Smoothie Bowl:

Start your day with a burst of antioxidants by blending a variety of berries with Greek yogurt, spinach, and a touch of honey. Top it with granola, nuts, and seeds for more texture and nutrients.

Berry Blast Smoothie Bowl:

Ingredients:

- ❖ 1 cup mixed berries (strawberries, blueberries, raspberries)

❖ 1/2 cup Greek yogurt

❖ Handful of spinach leaves

❖ 1 tablespoon honey

❖ Granola, nuts, and seeds for topping

Instructions:

❖ Blend mixed berries, Greek yogurt, spinach, and honey until smooth.

❖ Pour the smoothie into a bowl.

❖ Top with granola, nuts, and seeds for added crunch.

Benefits:

❖ High in antioxidants from berries.

❖ Greek yogurt provides protein.

❖ Spinach adds vitamins and minerals.

1.2 Green Goddess Power Smoothie:

Harness the power of leafy greens, such as kale and spinach, in this revitalizing smoothie. Combine with tropical fruits, chia seeds, and coconut water for a refreshing and nutrient-packed morning boost.

Green Goddess Power Smoothie:

Ingredients:

- ❖ 1 cup kale leaves
- ❖ 1 cup spinach leaves
- ❖ 1/2 cup pineapple chunks
- ❖ 1/2 cup mango chunks
- ❖ 1 tablespoon chia seeds
- ❖ Coconut water

Instructions:

- ❖ Blend kale, spinach, pineapple, mango, and chia seeds with coconut water.
- ❖ Blend until smooth.

Benefits

- ❖ Packed with leafy greens for vitamins and minerals.
- ❖ Chia seeds add fiber and omega-3 fatty acids.

1.3 Banana Almond Protein Smoothie:

Incorporate the creaminess of bananas and the protein punch of almond butter into this satisfying smoothie. Add a scoop of protein powder to get an extra protein boost.

Banana Almond Protein Smoothie:

Ingredients:

- ❖ 2 ripe bananas
- ❖ 2 tablespoons almond butter
- ❖ 1 cup almond milk
- ❖ 1 scoop protein powder (optional)

Instructions:

- ❖ Blend ripe bananas, almond butter, almond milk, and protein powder (if using).
- ❖ Blend until smooth.

Benefits:

- ❖ Bananas provide natural sweetness.
- ❖ Almond butter adds healthy fats and protein.

SECTION 2: ENERGIZING OAT CREATIONS:

2.1 Quinoa and Berry Breakfast Bowl:

Swap traditional oats for quinoa to create a protein-rich breakfast bowl. Top it with fresh berries, nuts, and a drizzle of honey for a wholesome and satisfying start to your day.

Quinoa and Berry Breakfast Bowl:

Ingredients:

- ❖ 1 cup cooked quinoa
- ❖ 1/2 cup mixed berries
- ❖ 2 tablespoons chopped nuts
- ❖ Drizzle of honey

Instructions:

- ❖ Combine cooked quinoa with mixed berries.
- ❖ Top with chopped nuts and a drizzle of honey.

Benefits:

- ❖ Quinoa offers protein and fiber.
- ❖ Berries provide antioxidants.

2.2 Overnight Chia Seed Pudding:

Prepare a nutritious and easy-to-digest chia seed pudding the night before. Customize with your favorite plant-based milk, fruits, and a sprinkle of cinnamon for added flavor.

Overnight Chia Seed Pudding:

Ingredients:

- ❖ 1/4 cup chia seeds
- ❖ 1 cup plant-based milk
- ❖ Mixed fruits
- ❖ Cinnamon for flavor

Instructions:

- ❖ Mix chia seeds with plant-based milk and let it sit in the refrigerator overnight.
- ❖ Top with mixed fruits and a sprinkle of cinnamon.

Benefits:

- ❖ Chia seeds are rich in omega-3 fatty acids.
- ❖ Plant-based milk adds calcium and vitamin D.

2.3 Warm Apple Cinnamon Oatmeal:

Embrace the comforting warmth of a classic oatmeal breakfast. Cook with diced apples, cinnamon, and a hint of nutmeg for a nourishing and heartwarming morning treat.

Warm Apple Cinnamon Oatmeal:

Ingredients:

- ❖ 1/2 cup rolled oats
- ❖ 1 apple, diced
- ❖ 1/2 teaspoon cinnamon
- ❖ Pinch of nutmeg

Instructions:

- ❖ Cook rolled oats with diced apples, cinnamon, and nutmeg.
- ❖ Stir until the oats are tender.

Benefits:

- ❖ Oats provide fiber and energy.
- ❖ Apples add natural sweetness.

Feel free to customize these recipes to your tastes and dietary needs. needs. Enjoy your nutritious breakfast!

SECTION 3: PROTEIN-PACKED BREAKFAST PLATES:

3.1 Avocado and Egg Toast:

Combine the creamy goodness of avocado with the protein boost of a poached egg on whole-grain toast. Sprinkle with chili flakes for an extra kick of flavor.

Avocado and Egg Toast:

Ingredients:

- ❖ 1 ripe avocado
- ❖ 1-2 eggs
- ❖ 2 slices of whole-grain bread
- ❖ Salt and pepper to taste
- ❖ Optional toppings: red pepper flakes, herbs, cherry tomatoes, feta, or hot sauce

Instructions:

Prepare Ingredients:

- ❖ Slice a ripe avocado and mash it in a bowl.

❖ Cook one or two eggs according to preference (poached, fried, or scrambled).

Toast Bread:

❖ Toast whole-grain bread slices until golden and crisp.

Assemble:

❖ Spread the mashed avocado evenly on the toasted bread.

Add Eggs:

❖ Place the cooked eggs on top of the mashed avocado.

Season:

❖ Sprinkle with salt, pepper, and any optional toppings you desire.

Serve:

❖ Enjoy the avocado and egg toast immediately while the bread is warm and the eggs are still runny.

Benefits:

Nutrient-Rich Combination:

- ❖ Avocado provides healthy monounsaturated fats, vitamins (C, E, K, B-6), and minerals (folate, potassium).
- ❖ Eggs contribute high-quality protein, vitamins (B-12, D), and essential nutrients (choline).

Heart-Healthy Fats:

- ❖ Monounsaturated fats in avocado support heart health by lowering bad cholesterol levels.

Protein-Packed:

- ❖ Eggs offer a complete protein source, aiding in muscle repair and maintenance.

Fiber Content:

- ❖ Whole-grain bread and avocado provide dietary fiber, supporting digestion and promoting satiety.

Satiety and Energy:

❖ The combination of healthy fats and protein promotes a feeling of fullness and sustained energy throughout the day.

Versatility:

❖ Customize with additional toppings like cherry tomatoes, feta, or a drizzle of hot sauce for added flavor and nutrients.

Quick and Nutrient-Dense:

❖ A quick and simple meal, ideal for busy mornings, providing a nutrient-dense start to the day.

Balanced Nutrition:

❖ The combination of fats, protein, and carbohydrates offers a balanced nutritional profile, suitable for a well-rounded meal.

Avocado and egg toast is a delicious, nutritious, and versatile option suitable for any meal. Its benefits extend beyond taste, providing a wholesome blend of essential nutrients for a satisfying and healthful experience.

3.2 Salmon and Cream Cheese Bagel:

Elevate your breakfast with a bagel topped with smoked salmon, cream cheese, and a sprinkle of capers. Rich in omega-3 fatty acids, this breakfast supports overall health.

Salmon and Cream Cheese Bagel:

Ingredients:

- 1 whole-grain bagel, sliced and toasted
- 4 oz smoked salmon
- 2 tbsp cream cheese
- Red onion, thinly sliced
- Capers (optional)
- Fresh dill for garnish
- Lemon wedges for serving

Instructions:

Prepare Bagel:

- Slice the whole-grain bagel and toast until golden.

Spread Cream Cheese:

- Spread cream cheese evenly on each half of the toasted bagel.

Layer Smoked Salmon:

❖ Arrange smoked salmon generously over the cream cheese.

Add Toppings:

❖ Place thinly sliced red onion rings on top of the salmon.

❖ Optionally, add capers for a burst of flavor.

Garnish:

❖ Sprinkle fresh dill over the assembled bagel for added freshness.

Serve:

❖ Serve the salmon and cream cheese bagel open-faced or as a sandwich.

❖ Accompany with lemon wedges on the side for a citrusy touch.

Benefits:

Omega-3 Fatty Acids:

❖ Salmon is rich in omega-3 fatty acids, supporting heart health and inflammation reduction.

High-Quality Protein:

- ❖ Salmon provides high-quality protein, essential for muscle repair and overall body function.

Creamy Texture and Flavor:

- ❖ Cream cheese adds a creamy texture and contributes to the overall rich and satisfying flavor.

Whole-Grain Nutrients:

- ❖ Whole-grain bagels offer fiber, vitamins, and minerals for sustained energy.

Antioxidant-Rich Garnish:

- ❖ Fresh dill not only enhances flavor but also provides antioxidants.

Low-Calorie Option:

- ❖ A satisfying and flavorful meal without excessive calories, suitable for a balanced diet.

Balanced Meal:

❖ The combination of protein, healthy fats, and carbohydrates creates a balanced and nutritious meal.

Quick and Elegant:

❖ Ideal for a quick and elegant breakfast or brunch, providing a sense of indulgence.

The Salmon and Cream Cheese Bagel offers a delightful combination of flavors and textures, making it a nutritious and enjoyable option for any time of the day.

3.3 Greek Yogurt Parfait:

Layer Greek yogurt with fresh fruits, granola, and a drizzle of honey to create a satisfying and protein-packed parfait. Add your favorite toppings for variety.

Greek Yogurt Parfait:

Ingredients:

❖ 1 cup Greek yogurt (unsweetened)
❖ 1/2 cup granola (choose a low-sugar option)

- ❖ 1/2 cup mixed berries (strawberries, blueberries, raspberries)
- ❖ 1 tablespoon honey (optional)
- ❖ 1 tablespoon nuts (almonds, walnuts) for topping
- ❖ Fresh mint leaves for garnish

Instructions:

Layer Greek Yogurt:

- ❖ In a glass or bowl, spoon a layer of Greek yogurt as the base.

Add Granola:

- ❖ Sprinkle a layer of granola over the Greek yogurt, creating a textural contrast.

Introduce Mixed Berries:

- ❖ Add a layer of mixed berries, distributing them evenly.

Repeat Layers:

- ❖ Repeat the layers until the glass or bowl is filled, ending with a final layer of berries on top.

Drizzle with Honey:

❖ Drizzle honey over the parfait for added sweetness, if desired.

Top with Nuts:

❖ Sprinkle nuts on the top layer for crunch and additional nutritional value.

Garnish with Mint:

❖ Garnish the parfait with fresh mint leaves for a burst of freshness.

Serve:

❖ Serve immediately and enjoy the layers of flavors and textures.

Benefits:

Protein-Packed Greek Yogurt:

❖ Greek yogurt is a rich source of protein, supporting muscle health and providing a feeling of fullness.

Nutrient-Dense Granola:

- ❖ Granola offers whole-grain goodness, providing fiber, vitamins, and minerals.

Antioxidant-Rich Berries:

- ❖ Mixed berries contribute antioxidants, promoting overall health and well-being.

Natural Sweetness with Honey:

- ❖ Honey adds a touch of natural sweetness while offering potential health benefits.

Healthy Fats from Nuts:

- ❖ Nuts provide healthy fats, adding satiety and a delightful crunch.

Digestive Health:

- ❖ The combination of yogurt and fiber-rich ingredients supports digestive health.

Versatility and Customization:

- ❖ Easily customizable with different fruits, nuts, or seeds based on personal preferences.

- ❖ The Greek Yogurt Parfait is a quick, nutritious, and satisfying option for a snack or breakfast.

Enjoy this delightful and nutritious Greek Yogurt Parfait as a flavorful and wholesome addition to your daily meals.

These breakfast boosters are more than just meals; they are nourishing rituals designed to provide essential nutrients and set a positive tone for your day. Experiment with these recipes, adjust them to your taste preferences, and embrace the joy of starting your mornings with delicious and healthful choices.

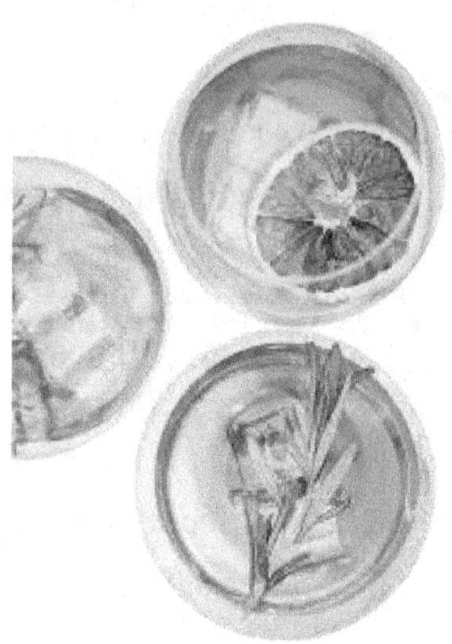

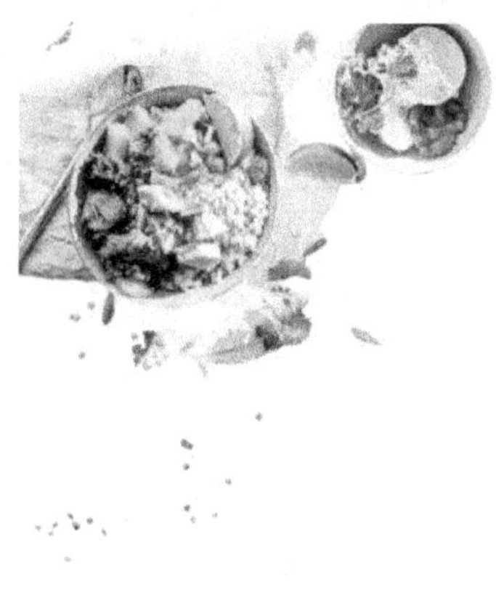

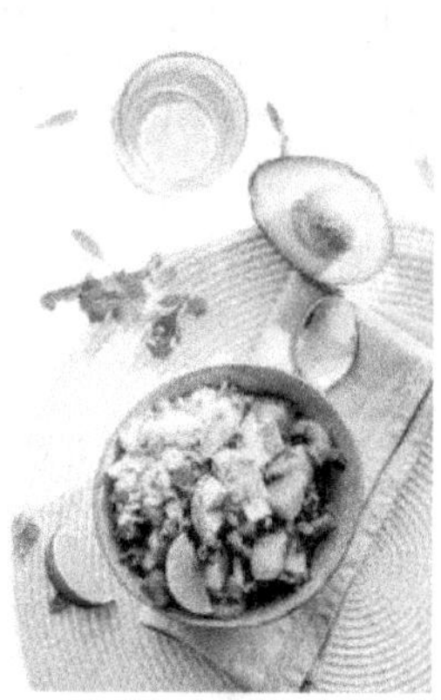

CHAPTER 3

SOUPS FOR HEALING.

In times of healing, a warm and nutrient-rich bowl of soup can be a source of comfort and nourishment. This chapter presents a collection of soothing soups designed to support your well-being and provide essential nutrients during your journey through cancer.

Healing Chicken and Vegetable Broth

Ingredients:

- ❖ 1 lb chicken, bone-in
- ❖ Assorted vegetables (carrots, celery, onion)
- ❖ 4 cups low-sodium chicken broth
- ❖ Fresh herbs (parsley, thyme)
- ❖ Salt and pepper to taste

Instructions:

- ❖ Simmer chicken, vegetables, and broth for 1-2 hours.
- ❖ Remove chicken, shred meat, and return to the broth.

- ❖ Season with fresh herbs, salt and pepper.

Benefits:

- ❖ Rich in collagen from chicken broth, aiding in tissue repair.
- ❖ Vegetables provide vitamins and minerals.

Butternut Squash and Ginger Soup

Ingredients:

- ❖ One medium butternut squash, peeled and diced
- ❖ 1 onion, chopped
- ❖ 2-inch piece of ginger, grated
- ❖ 4 cups vegetable broth
- ❖ Coconut milk (optional)
- ❖ Nutmeg, salt, and pepper to taste

Instructions:

- ❖ Sauté onion and ginger; add butternut squash and vegetable broth.
- ❖ Simmer until squash is tender; blend until smooth.

- ❖ Stir in coconut milk if desired, season with nutmeg, salt, and pepper.

Benefits:

- ❖ Butternut squash is rich in beta-carotene.
- ❖ Ginger offers anti-inflammatory properties.

Lentil and Spinach Healing Soup

Ingredients:

- ❖ 1 cup dried green lentils
- ❖ 1 onion, diced
- ❖ 2 carrots, sliced
- ❖ 2 cups fresh spinach
- ❖ 6 cups vegetable broth
- ❖ Cumin, coriander, salt, and pepper to taste

Instructions:

- ❖ Cook lentils, onion, and carrots in vegetable broth until tender.
- ❖ Add fresh spinach; season with cumin, coriander, salt, and pepper.

Benefits:

- ❖ Lentils provide protein and fiber.
- ❖ Spinach is a rich source of iron.

Miso and Mushroom Nourishing Soup

Ingredients:

- ❖ 4 cups mushroom broth
- ❖ 1 cup mixed mushrooms (shiitake, oyster)
- ❖ 3 tbsp miso paste
- ❖ Green onions, sliced
- ❖ Tofu cubes (optional)

Instructions:

- ❖ Simmer mushroom broth with mixed mushrooms.
- ❖ Dissolve miso paste in a ladle of hot broth; add to the pot.
- ❖ Garnish with green onions and tofu cubes if desired.

Benefits:

- ❖ Mushrooms contain immune-boosting properties.
- ❖ Miso provides probiotics for gut health.

Turmeric and Sweet Potato Comfort Soup

Ingredients:

- ❖ 2 sweet potatoes, peeled and diced
- ❖ 1 tsp turmeric powder
- ❖ 1 can coconut milk
- ❖ 4 cups vegetable broth
- ❖ Fresh cilantro for garnish
- ❖ Salt and pepper to taste

Instructions:

- ❖ Boil sweet potatoes with turmeric in vegetable broth until soft.
- ❖ Blend with coconut milk until smooth.
- ❖ Season with salt and pepper; garnish with fresh cilantro.

Benefits:

- ❖ Turmeric offers anti-inflammatory benefits.
- ❖ Sweet potatoes provide vitamins and fiber.

These healing soups are crafted with care to provide not only warmth but also essential nutrients to support your body's recovery. Allow their comforting flavors to bring solace and nourishment during your journey through cancer.

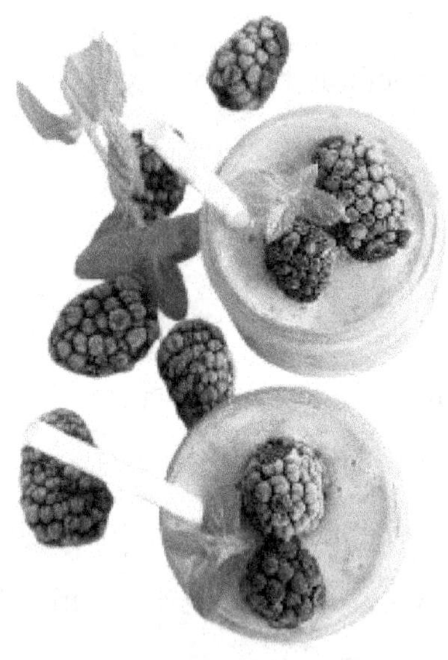

CHAPTER 4

SUPERCHARGED SALADS

Elevate your nutrition with vibrant and nutrient-packed salads. This chapter explores a variety of supercharged salads designed to provide a delicious and healthful boost during your journey through cancer. From leafy greens to colorful vegetables, these salads are a celebration of flavor and well-being.

Superfood Kale Salad with Citrus Vinaigrette

Ingredients:

- ❖ 4 cups chopped kale
- ❖ 1 cup quinoa, cooked
- ❖ 1 cup cherry tomatoes, halved
- ❖ 1 avocado, diced
- ❖ 1/4 cup pumpkin seeds
- ❖ Citrus vinaigrette (olive oil, lemon juice, honey)

Instructions:

- ❖ Massage kale with citrus vinaigrette.

- ❖ Toss kale with quinoa, cherry tomatoes, avocado, and pumpkin seeds.

Benefits:

- ❖ Kale is a nutrient powerhouse.
- ❖ Quinoa provides protein and fiber.
- ❖ Citrus adds vitamin C for immune support.

Colorful Beet and Goat Cheese Salad

Ingredients:

- ❖ 3 beets, roasted and sliced
- ❖ Mixed salad greens
- ❖ 1/2 cup goat cheese, crumbled
- ❖ 1/4 cup walnuts, chopped
- ❖ Balsamic vinaigrette dressing

Instructions:

- ❖ Arrange beets on a bed of mixed greens.
- ❖ Sprinkle with goat cheese and walnuts.
- ❖ Drizzle with balsamic vinaigrette.

Benefits:

- ❖ Beets offer antioxidants and fiber.
- ❖ Goat cheese adds protein and creaminess.

Quinoa and Chickpea Mediterranean Salad

Ingredients:

- ❖ 1 cup cooked quinoa
- ❖ 1 can chickpeas, drained
- ❖ Cherry tomatoes, halved
- ❖ Cucumber, diced
- ❖ Kalamata olives, sliced
- ❖ Feta cheese, crumbled
- ❖ Greek dressing

Instructions:

- ❖ Combine quinoa, chickpeas, tomatoes, cucumber, olives, and feta.
- ❖ Toss with Greek dressing.

Benefits:

- ❖ Quinoa and chickpeas provide protein.

❖ Mediterranean ingredients offer heart-healthy fats.

Asian-Inspired Edamame and Sesame Salad

Ingredients:

❖ 2 cups edamame, steamed

❖ Shredded red cabbage

❖ Carrots, julienned

❖ Bell peppers, thinly sliced

❖ Sesame seeds

❖ Soy-ginger dressing

Instructions:

❖ Mix edamame, cabbage, carrots, and bell peppers.

❖ Sprinkle with sesame seeds and toss with soy-ginger dressing.

Benefits:

❖ Edamame is a plant-based protein source.

❖ Sesame seeds add healthy fats.

Spinach and Berry Power Salad

Ingredients:

- ❖ 4 cups baby spinach
- ❖ Mixed berries (strawberries, blueberries)
- ❖ Goat cheese, crumbled
- ❖ Almonds, sliced
- ❖ Raspberry vinaigrette

Instructions:

- ❖ Combine spinach, berries, goat cheese, and almonds.
- ❖ Drizzle with raspberry vinaigrette.

Benefits:

- ❖ Spinach offers iron and vitamins.
- ❖ Berries provide antioxidants.

Supercharged salads are a delightful way to infuse your diet with essential nutrients and vibrant flavors. Embrace the diverse combinations presented in this chapter to nourish your body and enhance your well-being during your cancer journey.

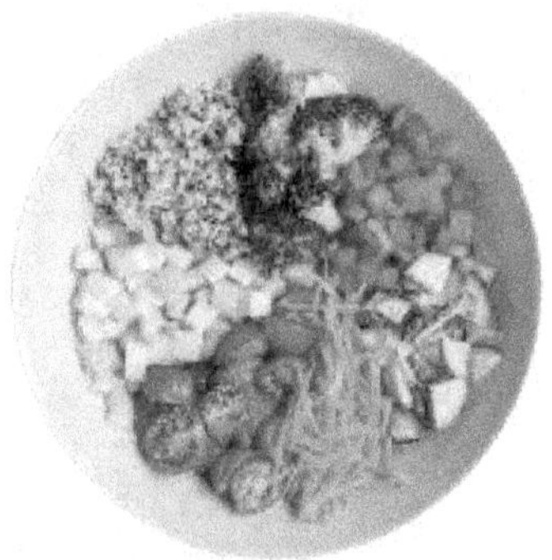

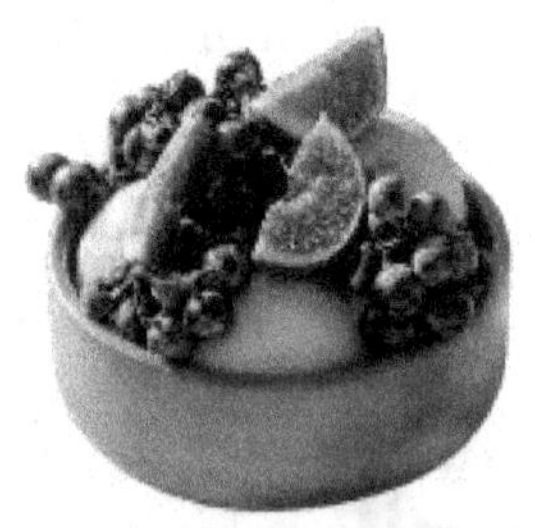

CHAPTER 5

POWERHOUSE PROTEINS

Fuel your body with strength and resilience through protein-packed dishes. This chapter is dedicated to providing a variety of recipes rich in high-quality proteins to support muscle maintenance and overall well-being during your journey through cancer. From lean meats to plant-based options, these powerhouse proteins are delicious and nutritious.

Grilled Salmon with Lemon-Herb Quinoa

Ingredients:

- ❖ Salmon fillets
- ❖ 1 cup quinoa, cooked
- ❖ Fresh herbs (parsley, dill)
- ❖ Lemon juice
- ❖ Olive oil
- ❖ Salt and pepper to taste

Instructions:

- ❖ Grill salmon until cooked.

❖ Mix cooked quinoa with fresh herbs, lemon juice, and olive oil.

❖ Serve salmon over the quinoa mixture.

Benefits:

❖ Salmon provides omega-3 fatty acids.

❖ Quinoa offers complete plant-based protein.

Chicken and Vegetable Stir-Fry

Ingredients:

❖ Chicken breast, sliced

❖ Mixed vegetables (broccoli, bell peppers, carrots)

❖ Soy sauce

❖ Garlic, minced

❖ Ginger, grated

❖ Brown rice, cooked

Instructions:

❖ Stir-fry chicken until cooked; set aside.

❖ Stir-fry vegetables with garlic and ginger.

❖ Combine chicken and vegetables; add soy sauce.

❖ Serve over cooked brown rice.

Benefits:

- ❖ Chicken is a lean source of protein.
- ❖ Vegetables add fiber and vitamins.

Lentil and Sweet Potato Curry

Ingredients:

- ❖ 1 cup dried lentils
- ❖ Sweet potatoes, diced
- ❖ Onion, chopped
- ❖ Coconut milk
- ❖ Curry powder
- ❖ Turmeric, cumin, coriander
- ❖ Fresh cilantro for garnish

Instructions:

- ❖ Cook lentils and sweet potatoes in coconut milk.
- ❖ Sauté onion; add curry powder, turmeric, cumin, and coriander.
- ❖ Mix lentils, sweet potatoes, and spiced onions.
- ❖ Garnish with fresh cilantro.

Benefits:

- ❖ Lentils provide plant-based protein.
- ❖ Sweet potatoes offer vitamins and fiber.

Quinoa and Black Bean Stuffed Peppers

Ingredients:

- ❖ Bell peppers, halved
- ❖ 1 cup quinoa, cooked
- ❖ Black beans, drained
- ❖ Corn kernels
- ❖ Salsa
- ❖ Taco seasoning
- ❖ Shredded cheese (optional)

Instructions:

- ❖ Mix quinoa, black beans, corn, salsa, and taco seasoning.
- ❖ Stuff peppers with the mixture.
- ❖ Bake until peppers are tender.Top with shredded cheese if desired.

Benefits:

- ❖ Quinoa and black beans offer a protein boost.
- ❖ Bell peppers provide vitamins and antioxidants.

Tofu and Vegetable Noodle Stir-Fry

Ingredients:

- ❖ Firm tofu, cubed
- ❖ Mixed vegetables (broccoli, snap peas, carrots)
- ❖ Rice noodles, cooked
- ❖ Soy sauce
- ❖ Sesame oil
- ❖ Garlic, minced

Instructions:

- ❖ Sauté tofu until golden.
- ❖ Stir-fry vegetables and garlic.
- ❖ Toss in cooked rice noodles, soy sauce, and sesame oil.

Benefits:

- ❖ Tofu is a plant-based protein source.
- ❖ Vegetables add vitamins and minerals.

Powerhouse proteins are essential for maintaining strength and vitality. Incorporate these diverse and flavorful recipes into your diet to ensure you're getting the protein your body needs during your cancer journey.

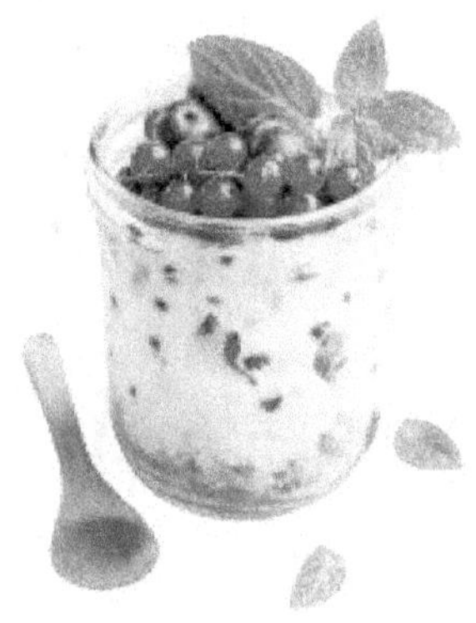

CHAPTER 6

SIDES WITH A PURPOSE

Complement your main dishes with sides that not only enhance flavor but also contribute essential nutrients. This chapter features versatile and purposeful side dishes, carefully curated to provide a well-rounded and satisfying dining experience during your journey through cancer.

Roasted Garlic and Herb Vegetables

Ingredients:

- ❖ Assorted vegetables (carrots, Brussels sprouts, potatoes)
- ❖ Garlic cloves, minced
- ❖ Fresh herbs (rosemary, thyme)
- ❖ Olive oil
- ❖ Salt and pepper to taste

Instructions:

- ❖ Toss vegetables with minced garlic, herbs, olive oil, salt, and pepper.

- ❖ Roast in the oven until brown and tender.

Benefits:

- ❖ Vegetables offer vitamins and fiber.
- ❖ Garlic adds immune-boosting properties.

Quinoa and Kale Pilaf

Ingredients:

- ❖ 1 cup quinoa, cooked\
- ❖ Kale leaves, chopped
- ❖ Lemon zest
- ❖ Almonds, sliced
- ❖ Olive oil
- ❖ Salt and pepper to taste

Instructions:

- ❖ Sauté the greens in olive oil until wilted.
- ❖ Mix with cooked quinoa, lemon zest, and sliced almonds.
- ❖ Season with salt and pepper.

Benefits:

- ❖ Quinoa provides protein and fiber.
- ❖ Kale offers vitamins and antioxidants.

Balsamic Glazed Brussels Sprouts

Ingredients:

- ❖ Brussels sprouts, halved
- ❖ Balsamic vinegar
- ❖ Honey
- ❖ Olive oil
- ❖ Salt and pepper to taste

Instructions:

- ❖ Roast Brussels sprouts until crisp.
- ❖ Mix balsamic vinegar, honey, and olive oil for glaze.
- ❖ Toss Brussels sprouts in the glaze; season with salt and pepper.

Benefits:

- ❖ Brussels sprouts are rich in antioxidants.
- ❖ Balsamic vinegar adds depth of flavor.

Lemon-Infused Asparagus Spears

Ingredients:

- ❖ Asparagus spears
- ❖ Lemon juice
- ❖ Olive oil
- ❖ Garlic powder
- ❖ Salt and pepper to taste

Instructions:

- ❖ Blanch asparagus in hot water.
- ❖ Drizzle with olive oil and lemon juice.
- ❖ Season with garlic powder, salt, and pepper.

Benefits:

- ❖ Asparagus provides vitamins and folate.
- ❖ Lemon adds a refreshing twist.

Turmeric and Coconut Cauliflower Rice

Ingredients:

- ❖ Cauliflower, grated
- ❖ Turmeric powder
- ❖ Coconut milk
- ❖ Fresh cilantro, chopped

* ❖ Salt and pepper to taste

Instructions:

* ❖ Sauté grated cauliflower with turmeric powder.
* ❖ Stir in coconut milk until cooked.
* ❖ Garnish with fresh cilantro, season with salt and pepper.

Benefits:

* ❖ Cauliflower is low in calories and high in fiber.
* ❖ Turmeric offers anti-inflammatory properties.

Sides with a purpose not only enhance the dining experience but also contribute vital nutrients to your overall well-being. Elevate your meals with these thoughtfully crafted side dishes, creating a balanced and satisfying culinary journey during your cancer recovery.

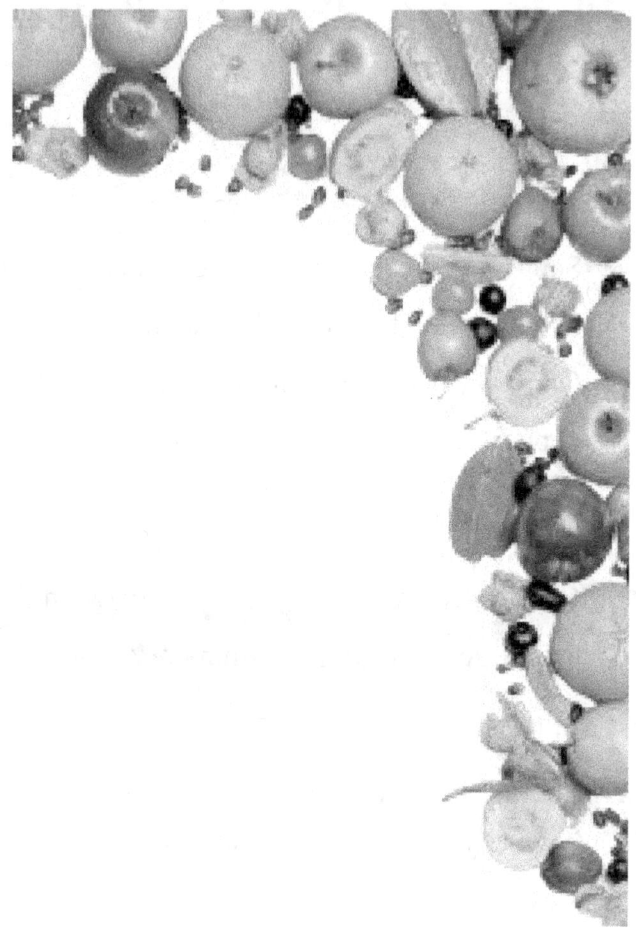

CHAPTER 7

HEALING BEVERAGES

Staying hydrated with purposeful and nourishing beverages is crucial during your cancer journey. This chapter explores a variety of healing beverages designed to soothe, hydrate, and provide essential nutrients. From comforting teas to rejuvenating smoothies, these beverages are crafted with your well-being in mind.

Ginger and Turmeric Immunity Elixir

Ingredients:

- ❖ Fresh ginger, grated
- ❖ Ground turmeric
- ❖ Honey
- ❖ Lemon juice
- ❖ Warm water

Instructions:

- ❖ Mix grated ginger and turmeric in warm water.
- ❖ Add honey and lemon juice to taste.
- ❖ Stir well and sip slowly.

Benefits:

- ❖ Ginger and turmeric have anti-inflammatory properties.
- ❖ Lemon adds vitamin C for immune support.

Soothing Herbal Chamomile Tea

Ingredients:

- ❖ Chamomile tea bag
- ❖ Hot water
- ❖ Honey (optional)
- ❖ Lemon slice (optional)

Instructions:

- ❖ Steep chamomile tea bag in hot water.
- ❖ Add honey and a lemon slice if desired.
- ❖ Enjoy the calming effects of chamomile.

Benefits:

- ❖ Chamomile promotes relaxation and aids digestion.
- ❖ Honey soothes the throat.

Berry and Spinach Detox Smoothie

Ingredients:

- ❖ Mixed berries (strawberries, blueberries)
- ❖ Fresh spinach leaves
- ❖ Greek yogurt
- ❖ Coconut water
- ❖ Chia seeds

Instructions:

- ❖ Blend berries, spinach, Greek yogurt, and coconut water.
- ❖ Add the chia seeds and mix until smooth.

Benefits:

- ❖ Berries provide antioxidants.
- ❖ Spinach adds vitamins and minerals.

Golden Milk Latte with Cinnamon

Ingredients:

- ❖ Turmeric latte mix
- ❖ Milk (dairy or plant-based)
- ❖ Cinnamon powder

- ❖ Maple syrup (optional)

Instructions:

- ❖ Mix turmeric latte mix with warm milk.
- ❖ Sprinkle with cinnamon.
- ❖ Sweeten with maple syrup if desired.

Benefits:

- ❖ Turmeric offers anti-inflammatory benefits.
- ❖ Cinnamon adds a warm and comforting flavor.

Green Tea Antioxidant Elixir

Ingredients:

- ❖ Green tea bag
- ❖ Hot water
- ❖ Fresh mint leaves
- ❖ Lemon wedge

Instructions:

- ❖ Steep green tea bag in hot water.
- ❖ Add fresh mint leaves and a lemon wedge.
- ❖ Enjoy the antioxidant-rich elixir.

Benefits:

- ❖ Green tea is high in antioxidants.
- ❖ Mint aids digestion and adds freshness.

Healing beverages play a vital role in supporting your overall well-being. Incorporate these soothing and nourishing drinks into your routine to stay hydrated and promote a sense of comfort and healing during your journey through cancer.

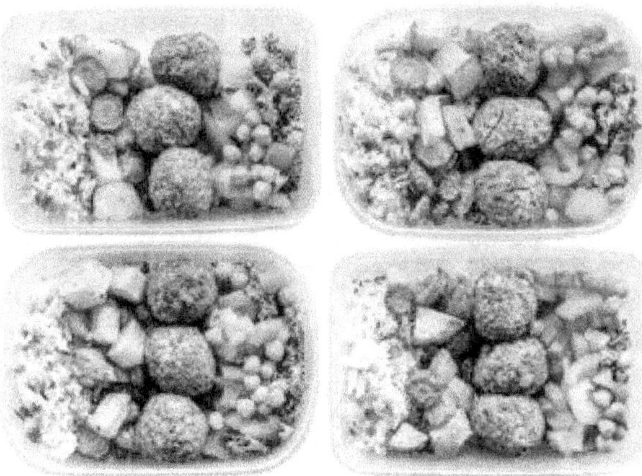

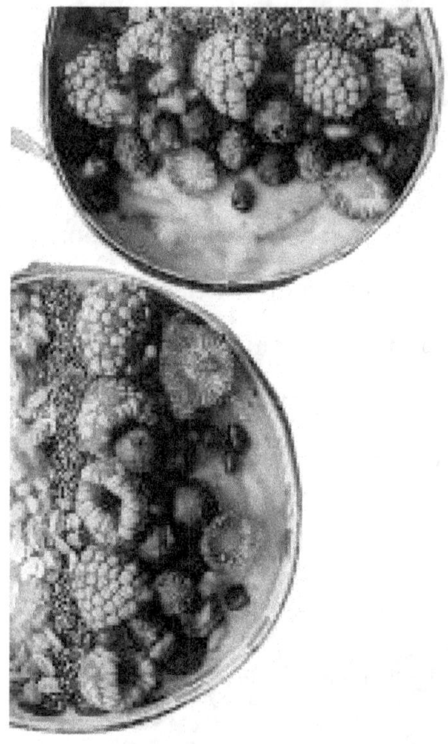

CHAPTER 8

SWEET INDULGENCES

Satisfy your sweet cravings with indulgent treats crafted to bring joy and comfort during your cancer journey. These sweet delights are not only delicious but also designed to incorporate wholesome ingredients that add a touch of sweetness without compromising on your health.

Dark Chocolate Avocado Mousse

Ingredients:

- ❖ Ripe avocados
- ❖ Dark chocolate, melted
- ❖ Cocoa powder
- ❖ Maple syrup
- ❖ Vanilla extract
- ❖ Fresh berries for garnish

Instructions:

- ❖ Blend avocados until smooth.

- ❖ Mix in melted dark chocolate, cocoa powder, maple syrup, and vanilla extract.
- ❖ Chill and serve topped with fresh berries.

Benefits:

- ❖ Avocado adds creaminess and healthy fats.
- ❖ Dark chocolate is rich in antioxidants.

Banana Nut Oat Cookies

Ingredients:

- ❖ Ripe bananas, mashed
- ❖ Rolled oats
- ❖ Chopped nuts (walnuts or almonds)
- ❖ Cinnamon
- ❖ Honey
- ❖ Vanilla extract

Instructions:

- ❖ Combine mashed bananas, oats, nuts, cinnamon, honey, and vanilla extract.
- ❖ Form cookies and bake till golden.

Benefits:

❖ Bananas offer natural sweetness.

❖ Oats provide fiber and sustained energy.

Berry Yogurt Parfait

Ingredients:

❖ Greek yogurt

❖ Mixed berries (strawberries, blueberries)

❖ Granola

❖ Honey

❖ Mint leaves for garnish

Instructions:

❖ Layer Greek yogurt with mixed berries and granola.

❖ Drizzle with honey and garnish with mint leaves.

Benefits:

❖ Greek yogurt adds protein.

❖ Berries provide antioxidants.

Coconut and Almond Energy Bites

Ingredients:

* ❖ Shredded coconut
* ❖ Almond flour
* ❖ Medjool dates, pitted
* ❖ Almond butter
* ❖ Vanilla extract
* ❖ Sea salt

Instructions:

* ❖ Blend shredded coconut, almond flour, dates, almond butter, vanilla extract, and a pinch of sea salt.
* ❖ Roll into bite-sized balls and chill.

Benefits:

* ❖ Dates add natural sweetness.
* ❖ Almond flour and butter offer protein and healthy fats.

Chia Seed Pudding with Fresh Mango

Ingredients:

- ❖ Chia seeds
- ❖ Coconut milk
- ❖ Maple syrup
- ❖ Vanilla extract
- ❖ Fresh mango, diced
- ❖ Shredded coconut for topping

Instructions:

- ❖ Mix chia seeds with coconut milk, maple syrup, and vanilla extract.
- ❖ Refrigerate until set; top with fresh mango and shredded coconut.

Benefits:

- ❖ Chia seeds provide omega-3 fatty acids.
- ❖ Fresh mango adds natural sweetness and vitamins.

Sweet indulgences can be a delightful part of your journey, bringing moments of joy and satisfaction. These treats are designed to be not only delicious but also nourishing, allowing you to enjoy the sweetness of life during your cancer recovery.

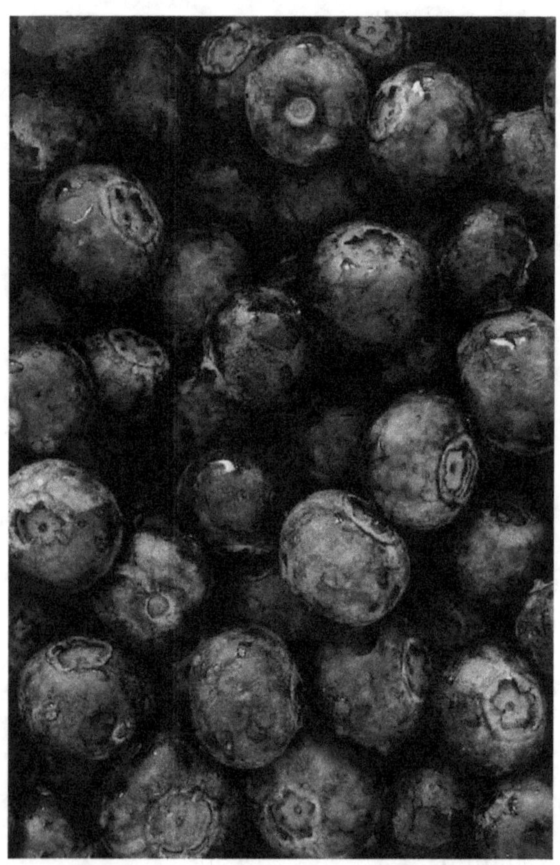

CHAPTER 9

CULINARY COMFORT FOR CHALLENGING TIMES

Navigating challenging times requires a special kind of nourishment that goes beyond the physical. This chapter offers a selection of comforting recipes designed to bring warmth, ease, and a sense of well-being during the difficult moments of your cancer journey. From soul-soothing soups to heartwarming dishes, these recipes are crafted with care to provide both physical and emotional comfort.

Homestyle Chicken and Rice Soup

Ingredients:

- ❖ Chicken thighs
- ❖ Carrots, celery, and onion, diced
- ❖ Chicken broth
- ❖ Basmati rice
- ❖ Fresh dill for garnish

Instructions:

- ❖ Simmer chicken with vegetables in chicken broth until cooked.
- ❖ Add basmati rice and continue simmering until rice is tender.
- ❖ Garnish with fresh dill before serving.

Benefits:

- ❖ Chicken provides protein.
- ❖ Basmati rice adds a comforting texture.

Creamy Butternut Squash Risotto

Ingredients:

- ❖ Butternut squash, diced
- ❖ Arborio rice
- ❖ Vegetable broth
- ❖ Parmesan cheese
- ❖ Nutmeg
- ❖ Fresh sage for garnish

Instructions:

- ❖ Sauté diced butternut squash and Arborio rice.
- ❖ Gradually add vegetable broth until rice is creamy.
- ❖ Stir in Parmesan cheese and a pinch of nutmeg.
- ❖ Garnish with fresh sage.

Benefits:

- ❖ Butternut squash is rich in vitamins.
- ❖ Arborio rice offers a creamy texture.

Comforting Macaroni and Cheese with Broccoli

Ingredients:

- ❖ Elbow macaroni
- ❖ Cheddar cheese, shredded
- ❖ Milk
- ❖ Butter
- ❖ Steamed broccoli florets
- ❖ Bread crumbs for topping

Instructions:

- ❖ Cook macaroni; drain and set aside.
- ❖ Make a cheese sauce with shredded cheddar, milk, and butter.
- ❖ Mix macaroni, cheese sauce, and steamed broccoli.
- ❖ Top with breadcrumbs and bake until golden.

Benefits:

- ❖ Broccoli adds vitamins and fiber.
- ❖ Cheese provides calcium and protein.

Lemon-Honey Glazed Baked Salmon

Ingredients:

- ❖ Salmon fillets
- ❖ Lemon juice
- ❖ Honey
- ❖ Garlic, minced
- ❖ Dijon mustard
- ❖ Fresh parsley for garnish

Instructions:

- ❖ Mix lemon juice, honey, minced garlic, and Dijon mustard.
- ❖ Coat salmon with the mixture and bake until flaky.
- ❖ Garnish with fresh parsley before serving.

Benefits:

- ❖ Salmon offers omega-3 fatty acids.
- ❖ Honey and lemon add a comforting glaze.

Vanilla Chai Rice Pudding

Ingredients:

- ❖ Arborio rice
- ❖ Chai tea
- ❖ Coconut milk
- ❖ Vanilla extract
- ❖ Cinnamon
- ❖ Raisins for sweetness

Instructions:

- ❖ Cook Arborio rice in chai tea and coconut milk.
- ❖ Stir in vanilla extract, cinnamon, and raisins.
- ❖ Simmer until rice is creamy and fully cooked.

Benefits:

- ❖ Chai tea adds aromatic spices.
- ❖ Coconut milk provides a rich and creamy base.

Culinary comfort is a powerful ally during challenging times. These recipes are crafted not just to nourish the body but also to provide a sense of solace and warmth. Embrace the comfort they bring and savor the moments of respite they offer during your cancer journey.

CONCLUSION

As we draw the curtain on the culinary journey that is "Nourishing Hope: A Cancer-Fighting Diet Cookbook," our hearts resonate with gratitude and a profound sense of purpose. In the realms of flavor and nutrition, we've not just explored recipes but forged a narrative of resilience, healing, and enduring hope.

This cookbook is more than a compilation of dishes; it stands as a testament to the transformative power of intentional nourishment. In every savory bite, we've discovered that a cancer-fighting diet is not just a menu but a love letter to the body—an affirmation of its incredible ability to rejuvenate, rebuild, and endure.

Each recipe etched onto these pages carries the whispers of countless stories—stories of battles waged with unwavering courage, of triumphs, and the quiet victories celebrated with every mindful mouthful. This cookbook is a celebration of mindful eating, where each forkful becomes a sacred act, a promise to cherish vitality, and a recognition of the sacredness inherent in every moment.

As we turn the last page, may you carry the essence of these recipes far beyond the kitchen. May the flavors linger in your daily life, infusing your journey with hope, resilience, and a deep-seated belief that nourishment is a steadfast ally on the path to healing. With every chop, simmer, and savoring moment, we hope you've not only found sustenance but a wellspring of strength and inspiration.

"Nourishing Hope" isn't just a cookbook; it's an invitation to continue this culinary expedition, not merely as a quest for delightful meals but as a celebration of life's extraordinary tapestry. May each dish serve as a vibrant brushstroke, painting a picture of health, hope, and enduring vitality.

As you journey forward, may each meal be a proclamation of your strength, each recipe a chapter in your story of triumph, and every bite a reminder that, with love, nourishment, and unyielding hope, you have the power to shape a narrative that inspires, uplifts, and nurtures the soul.

Here's to your ongoing journey—may your kitchen remain a sanctuary, and may each meal echo as a celebration of the remarkable tapestry that is your life. Until we meet again, may you savor the joys of nourishing hope.

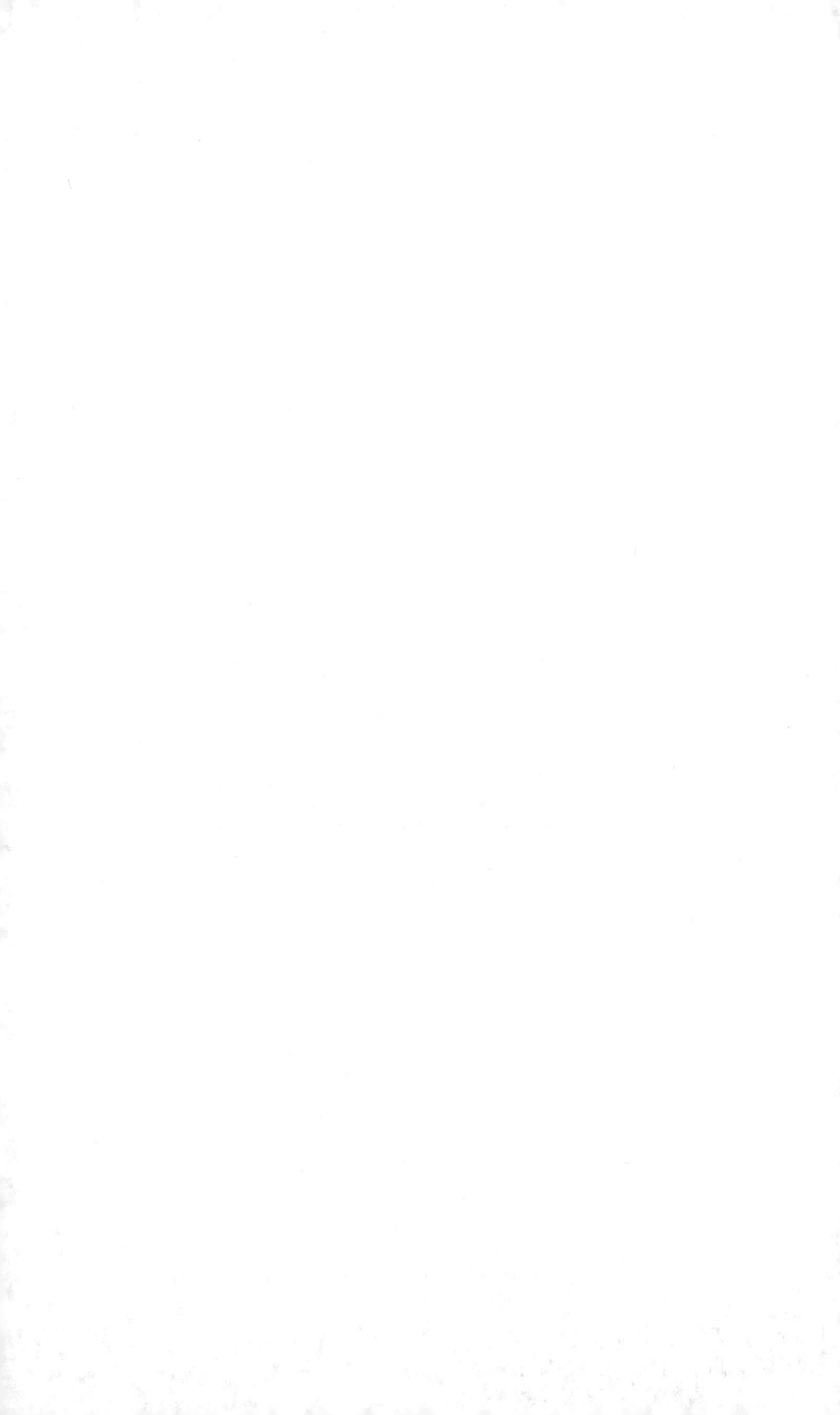